Contents

Fibromyalgia is a long-term (chronic) condition.

It causes:

- pain in the muscles and bones (musculoskeletal pain)

- areas of tenderness

- general fatigue

- sleep and cognitive disturbances

This condition can be hard to understand, even for healthcare providers. Its symptoms mimic those of other conditions, and there aren't any real tests to confirm the diagnosis. As a result, fibromyalgia is often misdiagnosed.

In the past, some healthcare providers even questioned whether fibromyalgia was real. Today, it is much better understood. Some of the stigma that used to surround it has eased.

BREAKFAST

1. Pan-Roasted Salmon with Lentil Pilaf

Prep Time: 15 mins

Cook Time: 40 mins

Total Time: 55 mins

Servings: 4

Ingredients

- 1 1/4 cup green lentils
- 1 dried bay leaf
- 3 Tbsp olive oil
- 1 large carrot diced (about 3/4 cup)
- 1/2 large onion chopped (about 3/4 cup)
- 1 rib celery diced (about 1/2 cup)
- 2 sprigs fresh thyme
- 1/2 tsp fennel seeds
- 1/4 tsp dried rosemary
- 1/2 cup dry red wine
- 4 fillets salmon with skin (about 5 oz each)

- 1/4 tsp dried thyme

- 1/2 juice of lemon (1 Tbsp plus 2 tsp)

- 1 tsp fresh thyme leaves

Instructions

1. Heat oven to 350°F. Bring 5 cups water to a boil in a medium saucepan on high heat. Add the lentils and bay leaf, reduce the heat to medium low, and simmer, partially covered, until the lentils are cooked through yet still firm to the bite, 20 to 22 minutes. Drain and discard the bay leaf.

2. Heat 1 Tbsp of the oil in a large skillet on medium heat. Add the carrot, onion, celery, thyme sprigs, fennel seeds, and rosemary. Cook, stirring occasionally, until the carrot is just tender, about 10 minutes. Add the wine and simmer until nearly evaporated, 3 to 4 minutes. Remove the thyme sprigs and bay leaf. Stir in the lentils and cook until heated through, about 1 minute. Season to taste with salt and freshly ground black pepper.

3. Heat the remaining 2 tsp of olive oil in a large ovenproof skillet on medium-high heat. Season the salmon with ¼

tsp salt and freshly ground black pepper. Rub the dried thyme between your fingers to crumble and rub over the salmon. Add to the skillet, flesh side down, and cook until golden brown, 2 to 3 minutes. Turn and sear skin, 1 minute. Transfer to the oven and roast until the flesh is opaque in the thickest part, 4 to 8 minutes, depending on thickness. Drizzle with the lemon juice and serve over the lentils. Garnish with the fresh thyme leaves.

2. Oatmeal Pecan Waffles (or Pancakes)

Prep Time: 10 mins

Cook Time: 30 mins

Total Time: 40 mins

Servings: 4

Ingredients

- 1 cup whole-wheat flour

- 1/2 cup quick-cooking oats

- 2 tsp baking powder

- 1 tsp sugar

- 1/4 cup unsalted pecans, chopped

- 2 large eggs, separated (for pancakes, see note)

- 1 1/2 cup fat-free (skim) milk

- 1 Tbsp vegetable oil

Fruit Topping

- 2 cups fresh strawberries, rinsed, stems removed and cut in half (or substitute frozen strawberries, thawed)

- 1 cup fresh blackberries, rinsed (or substitute frozen blackberries, thawed)

- 1 cup fresh blueberries, rinsed (or substitute frozen blueberries, thawed)

- 1 tsp powdered sugar

Instructions

1. Preheat waffle iron.

2. Combine flour, oats, baking powder, sugar and pecans in a large bowl.

3. Combine egg yolks, milk and vegetable oil in a separate bowl, and mix well.

4. Add liquid mixture to the dry ingredients, and stir together. Do not over mix; mixture should be a bit lumpy.

5. Whip egg whites into medium peaks. Gently fold egg whites into batter (for pancakes, see note below).

6. Pour batter into preheated waffle iron, and cook until the waffle iron light signals it's done or steam stops coming out of the iron. (A waffle is perfect when it is crisp and well-browned on the outside with a moist, light, airy and fluffy inside).

7. Add fresh fruit and a light dusting of powdered sugar to each waffle and serve.

3. Curry Scrambled Eggs

Prep Time: 5 mins

Cook Time: 15 mins

Total Time: 20 mins

Servings: 4

Ingredients

- 1 tablespoon avocado oil
- 2 cups leftover chicken breast or thighs, diced (you can substitute pre-cooked sausage, ham, or tofu if vegetarian)
- 1/4 onion, diced
- 1 cup mushrooms, diced
- 4 cups kale (or sub spinach or other greens work too)
- 6 eggs
- 1 tablespoon curry powder
- Salt and pepper to taste.

Instructions

1. Heat a large skillet over medium heat.

2. Add in the leftover chicken and onion. Cook for about 5 minutes, stirring occasionally.

3. While the chicken is cooking, crack your eggs into a medium bowl. Whisk with a fork until the eggs are mixed well.

4. Add in the kale and mushrooms to the skillet. Cook for another 5 minutes stirring occasionally.

5. Dump in the eggs and curry powder. Mix everything together well to get the curry powder all mixed in. Cook the eggs for a few minutes until they are no longer runny and are to your desired scrambled state.

6. Season with salt and pepper to taste.

7. Serve and enjoy your breakfast...or lunch...or dinner!

4. Homemade Pumpkin Bagels (Paleo, Gluten-Free)

Prep Time: 10 mins

Cook Time: 24 mins

Servings: 8

Ingredients

- Dry Ingredients:
- 1/3 cup coconut flour
- 3 tablespoon flaxseed meal
- 1 1/2 teaspoon pumpkin pie spice
- 1/2 teaspoon cinnamon
- Pinch of salt
- 1/2 teaspoon baking soda
- Wet Ingredients:
- 3 whole eggs
- 2 tablespoon coconut oil melted
- 1/4 cup non-dairy milk of choice (I used almond milk)

- 1/2 cup pumpkin puree

- 1 teaspoon vanilla extract

- 2 tablespoon maple syrup

- 1 teaspoon apple cider vinegar

Instructions

1. Preheat oven to 350°F and grease a donut or bagel pan.
2. In a bowl, add the dry ingredients, except for the baking soda, and mix until well combined.
3. In a separate bowl, add the wet ingredients, except for the apple cider vinegar, and mix until well combined.
4. In a small bowl, mix the apple cider vinegar and baking soda. Add this mixture to the wet ingredients.
5. Slowly add the dry mixture into the wet until well combined and the batter is smooth.
6. Pipe or spoon the batter into the prepared pan until all molds have an even amount of batter.
7. Bake for about 22-25 minutes or until a toothpick comes out clean. Remove from the oven and let sit for about 5 minutes before removing from the pan onto a cooling rack.

8. Serve and enjoy! Can be topped with ghee, nut butter, or
    even a chocolate spread!

5. Veggie Ranch Frittata

Prep Time: 10 mins

Cook Time: 20 mins

Total Time: 30 mins

Servings: 8

Ingredients

- 8 large eggs

- 1 red bell pepper, diced

- 1/2 a sweet onion, diced

- 1 cup kale

- 1/4 cup corn

- 1/4 cup black beans, rinsed, drained, & dried

- 1/3 cup shredded mozzarella cheese

- 1 teaspoon ranch seasoning, divided

- 1/2 tablespoon olive oil

- 1/4 teaspoon salt

- 1/4 teaspoon black pepper

Instructions

1. Preheat oven to 400.
2. Beat the eggs and combine with the mozzarella, salt, pepper, and 1/2 tsp ranch seasoning. Set aside.
3. Heat the olive oil in a well-greased cast iron skillet over medium heat. Spray the sides and the bottom of the skillet with some non-stick cooking spray to ensure eggs don't stick.
4. Once the oil is hot, add the onions and red pepper. Add a dash of salt to get the onions cooking down. Saute until the veggies are tender, approximately 5 minutes.
5. Add the kale, beans and corn to the skillet and cook for an additional 3-4 minutes until the kale is wilted and tender.
6. Add the other 1/2 tsp of ranch seasoning to the veggie mixture and stir.
7. Pour the egg mixture over top and very gently stir to move the veggies around a bit. Now leave it alone and let the edges of the egg mixture set. This will take just a few minutes.
8. Now move to the oven and bake for 15 minutes until it is cooked through.

9. Remove from the oven. Let cool on a wire rack for about
    5-10 minutes then slice and enjoy!

6. Mixed Mushroom Rice with Toasted Sesame Oil Sauce (Bibimbap)

Prep Time: 10 mins

Cook Time: 15 mins

Total Time: 25 mins

Servings: 3

Ingredients

- 8 ounces of mixed mushrooms (e.g., maitake, shitake, oyster, baby bella, enoki/washed, dried and roughly chopped)
- 12 garlic cloves (thinly sliced)
- 3 tablespoon extra virgin olive oil
- 1 heat of romaine lettuce (washed, dried and roughly chopped)
- 2 cups of cooked brown rice
- 4 tablespoon toasted sesame oil
- 4 teaspoon soy sauce
- 1/4 teaspoon sea salt
- ground pepper to taste
- 2 eggs (cooked)

Instructions

1. Sautee garlic with olive oil until soft.
2. Add mushrooms and sautee until cooked through, about 5-8 minutes, set aside.
3. Prepare sauce by mixing toasted sesame oil, soy sauce, sea salt and a pinch of ground pepper.
4. In a two bowls, evenly layer romaine lettuce, cooked rice, mushrooms.
5. Top each bowl with sunny side up eggs and sauce.
6. Mix and enjoy!

7. Dried Plum and Pistachio Chia Pudding

Prep Time: 5 mins

Cook Time: 60 mins

Total Time: 1 hour 5 mins

Ingredients

- 1/3 cup chia seeds
- 1 1/2 cups unsweetened almond milk (or other non-dairy milk)
- 1/2 cup California Dried Plums (chopped) + additional for topping
- 1/3 cup pistachios roasted + additional for topping
- 2 tablespoons hemp seeds
- 1 tablespoon cacao nibs unsweetened + additional for topping
- 2 teaspoon cinnamon ground

Instructions

1. Whisk together ingredients in large mixing bowl.
2. Cover and chill in fridge for at least one hour or overnight.
3. Once mixture reaches a pudding-like consistency, remove from fridge and divide into 2 bowls or mason jars.
4. Top with additional chopped California Dried Plums, pistachios, and cacao nibs before serving.

8. Honeynut Squash Yogurt Parfait (Gluten-Free)

Prep Time: 5 mins

Cook Time: 25 mins

Total Time: 30 mins

Servings: 4

Ingredients

- 4 honeynut squash (or sweet potatoes)
- coconut oil spray
- 1/2 teaspoon ground cinnamon
- 4 teaspoon coconut sugar
- 4 teaspoon maple syrup (optional)
- 1 cup of yogurt
- 4 scoop of Further Food Vanilla Collagen
- 1/2 cup of homemade gluten-free granola
- 4 tablespoon of maple almond butter

Instructions

1. Preheat oven to 375F and line a baking sheet with parchment paper
2. Cut off the top of the squash, then cut in half lengthwise and scoop out seeds
3. Spray with coconut oil then sprinkle with ground cinnamon and coconut sugar
4. Drizzle with some maple syrup too (optional)
5. Lay face down on a baking sheet and bake for 25-30 min, or until softened
6. Honeynut is a sweeter squash, but you could also use a sweet potato!
7. Serve with yogurt (I did plain mixed with Further Food vanilla collagen), homemade granola, and maple almond butter.

9. Asparagus and Feta Frittata (Vegetarian, Gluten-Free)

Prep Time: 10 mins

Cook Time: 45 mins

Total Time: 55 mins

Servings: 6

Ingredients

- 8 eggs

- 1/2 cup half-and-half (use coconut milk for dairy-free)

- 1/2 cup diced yellow onion

- 3 garlic cloves, minced

- 2 tablespoons olive oil

- 2 teaspoons salt

- 1/4 teaspoon black pepper

- 1 teaspoon garlic powder

- 6 ounces feta cheese

- 1 pound fresh asparagus

Instructions

1. Preheat oven to 400 degrees F.

2. Chop ends off washed asparagus. Cut 1/3 of the asparagus into bite-sized pieces, leaving the rest whole. With the whole asparagus, toss with olive oil, salt, and pepper, and set aside.

3. Stovetop, turn a pan onto medium heat and add olive oil once warmed.

4. Add diced yellow onion, minced garlic, chopped asparagus, and a pinch of salt to the pan, stirring and cooking for approximately 5 minutes.

5. In a large bowl, crack eggs and whisk well.

6. Add half-and-half, salt, pepper, garlic powder, and almost all of the feta to the bowl. Set aside remaining feta.

7. In a 9×9 oven-safe square or round baking dish, add the asparagus-onion-garlic mixture to the bottom and spread evenly around the dish.

8. Pour the egg-milk-cheese mix over the veggies and spread evenly.

9. Bake for about 15 minutes, or until eggs are somewhat set, remove from oven, and add the asparagus spears on top of the frittata in a line.
10. If the asparagus start to sink, cook the frittata for a few more minutes before adding.
11. Finish baking for about 15-25 more minutes.
12. Check doneness by inserting a toothpick into the frittata. If there is no residue (and no jiggly eggs), it is done.
13. Serve warm and top with remaining feta cheese and cracked black pepper.

10. Spinach and Fresh Herb Frittata

Prep Time: 10 mins

Cook Time: 40 mins

Total Time: 50 mins

Servings: 6

Ingredients

- 8 extra large Free Range Eggs
- 1/2 cup nut milk of choice
- 5 Spring Onions, finely choppe
- 1 cup Baby Spinach, chopped
- 1 cup Sweet Cherry Tomatoes, quartered
- 1 cup Fresh Flat Leaf Parsley, chopped
- 1 cup Fresh Cilantro, chopped
- 4 cloves Garlic, minced
- 3 tablespoons Fresh Chives, finely chopped
- Pinch Himalayan Pink Salt
- Generous amount of Black Pepper
- 4 tablespoons Almond Meal

Instructions

1. Pre-heat fan-forced oven to 350°F.
2. In a large bowl whisk eggs lightly with nut milk.
3. Add spring onions, spinach, tomatoes, herbs, garlic, chives, salt and pepper and mix well.
4. Add almond meal and mix to combine.
5. Pour over egg mixture into a greased quiche dish.
6. Bake in oven for 35-40 minutes or until egg is set.
7. Serve warm or chilled.

11. Honey Walnut Shrimp with Rainbow Slaw

Prep Time: 20 mins

Cook Time: 20 mins

Total Time: 40 mins

Servings: 2

Ingredients

- 1/8 cup raw sugar or coconut sugar
- 1/4 cup water
- 1/2 cup raw walnuts
- 1/4 cup avocado oil mayonnaise
- 2 tablespoons full-fat coconut milk, canned
- 2 tablespoons honey raw, local if possible
- 1/2 cup tapioca flour
- 12 shrimp deveined, peeled, thawed
- 1 teaspoon salt
- 1/4 teaspoon garlic powder
- 1/4 cup coconut oil

- 1 cup rice organic brown or white, cooked
- 2 carrots, shaved
- 1/2 of a red bell pepper, mandolined
- 1/4 of a large head of cabbage, mandolined
- 1 tablespoon sesame oil
- 1 tablespoon coconut aminos sub soy sauce for non-GF
- 1/2 of a lime, juiced

Instructions

1. Preheat oven to 350 degrees F.
2. Mix the sugar and water in a small saucepan and bring to a boil.
3. Once at a boil, turn off heat and add walnuts. Coat walnuts with the syrup.
4. Spread walnuts on a parchment-paper-lined baking sheet without touching each other; bake for 8-10 minutes.
5. In a small bowl, whisk the mayo, coconut milk, and honey. Set aside.
6. In a large Ziploc bag, add the tapioca flour, shrimp, salt, and garlic powder.
7. Shake to coat the shrimp evenly and well.

8. In a large pan, heat up the coconut oil and add the battered shrimp, in bathes if needed.

9. Cook the shrimp 3-4 minutes per side. Check for golden brown crispiness before flipping.

10. Serve over cooked rice and generously add the creamy honey sauce.

11. For the rainbow slaw salad: Grate carrots with a vegetable peeler and mandolin the bell pepper and the cabbage into thin strips. Mix with sesame oil, coconut aminos/soy sauce, and lime juice. Mix well.

12. Cassava Flour Breaded Buffalo Chicken

Prep Time: 1 hour

Cook Time: 20 mins

Total Time: 1 hour 20 mins

Servings: 4

Ingredients

- 2 lbs chicken breast
- 1 egg
- ½ cup coconut milk
- 1 cup cassava flour
- 1 teaspoon paprika
- 1 tablespoon garlic salt
- 1 tablespoon onion powder
- 2 teaspoons avocado oil
- 4 tablespoons buffalo sauce

Instructions

1. Whisk egg and milk together in a large bowl. Place all of your chicken into the bowl, ensuring it is all covered. Place the bowl in the fridge for at least 1 hour.
2. Heat a pan on the stove over medium heat with avocado oil for about five minutes or until warm.
3. While the pan is heating, mix together cassava flour, paprika, garlic salt and onion powder in a large bowl and place next to the stove.
4. Remove the chicken from the refrigerator and place the bowl next to the cassava flour mixture.
5. Piece by piece, move chicken from the milk to the flour using a fork and cover completely.
6. Carefully transfer the chicken to the stove and cook for 5-7 minutes on each side. Tip: if the bottom of your pan is coated in excess flour after cooking a batch, clean out pan and start the oil heating step again to achieve clean, not burnt chicken.
7. Move the chicken to a drying rack and let cool so that the coating is less likely to fall off.
8. Once chicken cools a bit, coat with buffalo sauce.
9. Enjoy!

13. Vegetarian Curry Soup

Prep Time: 5 mins

Cook Time: 15 mins

Total Time: 20 mins

Servings: 4

Ingredients

- 1/2 onion, diced

- 2 large carrots peeled, diced

- 1 can garbanzo beans chickpeas

- 1/2 cup frozen peas

- 3 tablespoon olive oil

- 1 can lite coconut milk

- 1/3 cup vegetable stock

- 1 tablespoon arrowroot

- 1 tablespoon coconut sugar

- 1 tablespoon curry powder

- 1 tablespoon fresh lime juice

- 1 teaspoon dried basil

- 1 teaspoon minced garlic

- Salt & Black Pepper

Instructions

1. Combine the coconut milk, arrowroot powder, and coconut sugar. Stir well until there are no clumps, and set to the side.

2. Heat the olive oil over medium heat. Once the pan is hot, add the diced carrots, onions and some salt and pepper. Cook for about 7-8 minutes or until carrots are tender and onions are translucent.

3. To the carrots and onions, add the garbanzo beans, green peas, dried basil, curry powder and minced garlic. Stir and cook for 1-2 more minutes. Add a little more sea salt and ground black pepper to season the beans and peas.

4. Add the vegetable stock to the veggie/bean mixture and warm everything together.

5. Now add the coconut milk mixture stirring constantly until warmed and combined.

6. Simmer for 5-7 minutes. The soup will begin to thicken, and then it's done!

7. Finish by mixing in the fresh lime juice. Enjoy!

14. Marinated Citrus Ginger Tofu Soba Noodle Salad (vegan, gluten-free)

Prep Time: 20 mins

Cook Time: 30 mins

Total Time: 50 mins

Servings: 4

Ingredients

For the tofu:
- 2 tablespoons orange juice
- 2 tablespoons tamari or soy sauce
- 2 tablespoons sesame oil
- 2 tablespoons olive oil
- 1 teaspoon honey
- 1 teaspoon grated ginger
- 2 teaspoon grated or minced garlic
- 1 package firm or extra firm tofu (cut into 1 inch cubes)

For the Salad:
- 4 ounces buckwheat soba noodles
- 2 teaspoon lime juice

- 2 tablespoons orange juice

- 3 tablespoons rice vinegar

- Leftover liquid from tofu bake, above

- 1 stalk broccoli (florets only, cut small)

- 1 large carrot (cut into small matchsticks)

- 1 cup snow peas

- 1 cup chopped lacinato kale

- 1/3 cup cilantro (chopped)

Instructions

1. Preheat the oven to 350 degrees.
2. In a bowl mix orange juice, tamari/soy sauce, sesame oil, olive oil, honey, ginger, garlic.
3. Place tofu in oven safe baking dish and pour mixture over tofu.
4. Put the tofu into the oven and bake for 15 minutes, stir, and bake for 15 minutes more, or until browned.
5. Remove from oven and set aside to cool.
6. Pour remaining liquid from baking dish into a bowl.
7. To prepare salad, boil the soba noodles based on package instructions and rinse with cold water when done.

8. Meanwhile, add lime juice, orange juice, rice vinegar to the baking liquid and set aside.

9. In a large bowl combine cooked noodles, broccoli, carrots, snow peas, kale, cilantro, tofu and toss with the dressing mixture.

15.Quick & Easy Tempeh Taco Bowl

Prep Time: 10 mins

Cook Time: 8 mins

Total Time: 18 mins

Servings: 2

Ingredients

- 1 package of organic tempeh

- 1 tablespoon avocado oil

- 1/2 cup sweet onion, chopped

- 1 tablespoon of your favorite taco spice blend

- Bowl toppings:
- Mixed greens

- Bell peppers

- Black beans

- Avocado

- Tomatoes

- Corn

- Cucumbers

- Salsa

- Cilantro

Instructions

1. In a skillet or fry pan sauté the onions with the oil over medium heat until translucent.
2. Crumble the tempeh and add it to the pan along with the spice blend. If the mixture seems to dry you can add additional oil.
3. Once the mixture is warmed through remove from the heat.
4. Slice/chop/prep your bowl ingredients and place into containers for storing along with the tempeh mixture.
5. Enjoy right away or store for up to 5 days in the fridge for a healthy lunch or dinner that's ready to go!

16. Healthy Crockpot White Chicken Chili

Prep Time: 30 mins

Total Time: 6-8 hours

Serving: 8

Ingredients

- 2-3 large boneless skinless chicken breasts
- 2 15.5 ounce cans of reduced sodium great northern beans (drained and rinsed)
- 1-15 ounce of sweet golden corn (drained and rinsed)
- 1-4.5 ounce can of chopped green chiles
- 2-14.5 ounce cans reduced sodium chicken broth
- 1 medium sweet yellow onion (chopped)
- 3 garlic cloves (minced)
- 1 lime (juiced)
- 1 teaspoon cumin
- 1/2 teaspoon onion powder
- 1/2 teaspoon garlic powder
- 1 1/2 teaspoon chili powder
- 1/4 teaspoon cayenne pepper

- black pepper (to taste)
- paprika (to taste)
- Optional: Superfood Turmeric, plain Greek yogurt, chunky salsa, and reduced fat
- shredded cheese for topping

Instructions

1. Place chicken breasts, Great Northern beans, corn, green chilies, chopped onion, minced garlic, and spices in the crockpot.
2. Add two cans of chicken broth and squeeze the juice of one lime over the mixture.
3. Cook on low for 6 to 8 hours.
4. Before removing from crockpot, use two forks to shred the chicken. Stir ingredients thoroughly.
5. Serve with toppings as desired. I enjoyed mine with crushed multigrain tortilla chips, plain Greek yogurt, reduced fat shredded cheese, and hot salsa!

17. Chickpea Pasta with Mushroom Goat Cheese Sauce

Prep Time: 10 mins

Cook Time: 20 mins

Total Time: 30 mins

Servings: 4

Ingredients

- on 8 oz dry macaroni shaped pasta (Banza chickpea pasta)

- 8 oz cremini mushrooms

- 1 tablespoon ghee

- 6 oz goat cheese

- 2 cups spinach

- 1/2 cup bone broth

- 1 teaspoon salt

- 1/8 teaspoon black pepper

- 1/4 teaspoon garlic powder

- 1 tablespoon tapioca flour

- 1 tablespo water

Instructions

1. Boil water for pasta and cook to package instructions.

2. Heat up bone broth in small saucepan until warm.

3. Blend or puree bone broth and goat cheese; add back to saucepan.

4. Add salt, pepper, garlic powder and a tapioca slurry (tapioca flour mixed with water) to thicken. Stir sauce often, until it becomes thick.

5. Meanwhile, saute mushrooms in ghee and add salt for about 10 minutes. Add spinach at the end and mix well until wilted.

6. Add pasta, mushrooms and spinach mixture, and goat cheese into a large pot and mix well together.

18. Roasted Cabbage with Crispy Chickpeas and Tahini Sauce (Vegan)

Prep Time: 15 mins

Cook Time: 40 mins

Total Time: 55 mins

Servings: 4

Ingredients

For the cabbage:

- 1 small to medium red cabbage (any type of cabbage can be used)

- Extra virgin olive oil

- Salt and pepper

- 1/4 teaspoon fennel seeds

- 1/4 teaspoon dry dill

- For the chickpeas:
- 1 heaping cup pressure cooked chickpeas (drained)

- 4-6 spring onions, chopped

- 1 garlic clove, finely sliced

- salt and pepper

- For the tahini sauce:
- 2 tablespoons tahini paste

- 1/2 teaspoon lemon juice

- 1/4 tsp raw, local honey

- Few teaspoons cold water (added one by one until you get the desired consistency)

Instructions

1. Preheat the oven to 400F (200C).
2. Wash and cut the cabbage in wedges, the number will depend on how big your cabbage is. The sugar loaf cabbage I used is pretty small so I had four wedges.
3. Add the cabbage to a baking dish, drizzle with extra virgin olive oil, sprinkle with salt and pepper and dry dill and roast for 35-40 minutes. You can add a little water in the last 15 minutes if it looks to dry.
4. Add the cooked chickpeas to another baking dish that will fit next to the cabbage, add the onions and garlic, sprinkle with salt and pepper, drizzle with olive oil,

toss and put in the oven. It will need about 35 minutes to get crispy (they are not totally crispy, but pretty dry compared to the boiled ones).

5. While the veggies are cooking, make the tahini sauce. Add the tahini to a small bowl with the lemon juice and honey, start mixing, preferably with a mini hand mixer, or a fork and start adding cold water, one teaspoon at a time, and continue until it becomes creamy and easy to drizzle, but the consistency is up to you. If the tahini is not salted, taste and see if it needs a pinch of salt.

6. When the cabbage and chickpeas are ready, add the cabbage wedges to a serving platter, spread the chickpeas on top, drizzle the tahini sauce and sprinkle fresh dill. If everything is well seasoned you won't need extra salt, but if it needs more add some.

19. Thai Beef Coconut Noodles

Prep Time: 20 mins

Cook Time: 1 hour

Total Time: 1 hour 20 mins

Servings: 6

Ingredients

- skirt steak (20 ounces)
- 1/2 cup coconut milk
- 3 tablespoons gluten free soy sauce
- 1 teaspoon ginger (grated)
- 2 teaspoons fish sauce
- 1 package glass rice noodles
- 1/4 cup peanuts
- 1/4 cup snap peas
- 1/4 cup mung
- 1/4 cup bean sprouts
- 1/4 cup star anise
- 1/2 teaspoon cumin
- 1 teaspoon garlic

- 1/2 teaspoon coriander
- optional: include chili's in marination

Instructions

1. Marinate steak in chilis, ginger, soy, fish sauce and rice vinegar for 20 minutes .
2. Then slice beef into bits ans fry it off until it's cripsy with the peanuts.
3. Put beef aside and place into pan garlic, chillis, ginger on medium heat.
4. Add in fish and soy sauce for 15 minutes with the peas.
5. Once cooked but not overcooked add the beef and peanuts , coconut milk and noodles and cook for 5 minutes to get all the flavors working together.
6. Add in mung bean sprouts and a hefty amount of chopped coriander to finish

20. Massaged Kale Salad with Chicken

Prep Time: 20 mins

Cook Time: 15 mins

Total Time: 35 mins

Servings: 6

Ingredients

Chicken Marinade Ingredients:

- 1 pound boneless, skinless chicken breast
- 1/4 cup apple cider vinegar
- 3 cloves garlic, minced
- 1/4 cup olive oil
- 1 tablespoon fresh thyme or 1 teaspoon dried thyme
- 1/2 teaspoon salt

Salad Ingredients:

- 1 bunch kale, about 8 cups, chopped or ripped into bite-sized pieces
- 2 cups squash or potato of your choice (sweet potato, butternut squash, delicata squash, or acorn squash), cut into 1/2-inch cubes

- 1/4 cup pecans
- 1 apple of your choice, julienned (any variety you like)
- 1 cup cooked quinoa
- 1/4 cup crumbled goat cheese or feta cheese
- Apple Cider Vinaigrette Ingredients:
- 1/2 cup olive oil
- 3 tablespoons apple cider vinegar
- 3 tablespoons dijon mustard
- 3 tablespoons maple syrup
- 1/4 teaspoon salt

Instructions

1. Combine all chicken marinade ingredients in a large zip top bag or container and let marinate for 20 minutes up to 2 hours.
2. While waiting for the chicken to marinate, combine all vinaigrette ingredients in a mason jar or tupperware. Shake vigorously until combined.
3. Add kale to a large salad bowl. Pour ¼ cup of prepared vinaigrette over kale. Using both hands, massage kale for 2-3 minutes until kale feels softer and reduces down by about half.

4. Heat two separate skillets over medium-high heat. Coat squash or potato in 2 tablespoons vinaigrette then add to one of the skillets. Sautee for about 15 minutes, or until tender and lightly browned.

5. At the same time, remove chicken from marinade and add into the other skillet. Cook chicken 5 to 6 minutes on one side without moving it around. Then, flip chicken and cook for 8 more minutes, or until internal temperature reaches 165° F.

6. Top kale with cooked squash or potato, chicken, pecans, apple, quinoa, and crumbled goat cheese. Drizzle with more vinaigrette as desired and enjoy!

21. Salmon Burgers with Cilantro Avocado Sauce

Prep Time: 15 mins

Cook Tmie: 30 mins

Total Time: 45 mins

Servings: 4

Ingredients

- 1 lb wild caught salmon
- 1/2 cup bread crumbs (*I used sprouted crackers, turn into bread crumbs w/ food processor)
- 1/4 cup onion, chopped
- 1/2 cup parsley, chopped
- few pinches of sea salt (or to preference)
- few pinches of pepper (or to preference)
- 3 heaping tablespoons Dijon Mustard
- juice of 1 lime
- 1 egg

Cilantro Avocado Sauce:

- 1/2 cup cilantro leaves, chopped

- 1 whole avocado

- 1/2 teaspoon pink himalayan sea salt (or to taste)

- pepper   to   taste

  1/2 cup olive oil (*or more to thin to desired to consistency)

- juice of 1 lime

Instructions

1. Pre-heat the oven to 375 degrees and line a baking sheet with parchment paper. Set aside.

2. Side note: If you only have one food processor, like me! make the sauce first, so you don't have to completely wash it out after using it for the raw fish.

3. Over medium heat, add 1 tbsp. coconut oil or olive oil to a sauce pan and cook the onion until fragrant/tender. Roughly 5-7 minutes. Set aside and allow to cool.

4. In a large mixing bowl, add the beaten egg and the salmon burger ingredients except for the salmon to the bowl.

5. For the salmon. I buy 1 pd. of wild salmon, therefore I have to take the skin off. I then, add the salmon into chunks, into my food processor and pulse it a few times. The consistency will be chunky, be careful to not over process and pulse where it turns into a pate or mush. You want it to hold together.

6. Add the salmon to the bowl and mix thoroughly.

7. Separate the mixture into four even patties and place in the parchment paper. Bake at 375 for 12 minutes on one side THEN flip, bake for an additional 8-10 minutes on the opposite side.

8. Serve in on patties, in a pita, on tacos with the sauce! The burgers will stay fresh for up to three days or freeze them for the longer!

9. For the Cilantro Avocado Sauce:

10. Combine all the ingredients in your food processor or blender and mix until creamy. Taste test and adjust to preference. Makes one 1 cup or so and will last about 1 week in fridge.

22. One Pan Lemon & Thyme Chicken Milanese

Prep Time: 1 hour 10 mins

Cook Time: 30 mins

Total Time: 1 hour 40 mins

Servings: 4

Ingredients

- 4 chicken breasts

- 1 egg

- ½ cup milk

- ½ cup cassava flour

- 1 teaspoon paprika

- 1 tablespoon garlic salt

- 1 tablespoon onion powder

- 1 cup cherry tomatoes

- 2 tablespoons garlic, minced

- 1 shallot, diced

- 3 tablespoons fresh thyme

- 1 lemon, juiced

- ¼ cup fresh basil

- 4 tablespoons avocado oil, separated in half

- ½ cup ghee, separated in half

Instructions

1. Whisk egg and milk together in a large bowl. Place all of your chicken into the bowl, ensuring it is all covered then sprinkle salt and pepper over top. Place the bowl in the fridge for at least 1 hour.

2. Heat a pan on the stove over medium heat with 2 tbsp avocado oil for about five minutes or until warm.

3. Once warm, add in tomatoes, shallot, garlic and 2 tbsp of the thyme. Sauté for about 5 minutes. While cooking, mix together cassava flour, paprika, garlic salt and onion powder in a large bowl and place next to the stove.

4. Transfer the tomato mixture to a plate and remove the chicken from the refrigerator. Place the bowl next to the cassava flour mixture and add ¼ cup ghee and 2 tbsp

avocado oil back into your skillet. Let heat until simmering.

5. Piece by piece, move chicken from the milk to the flour using a fork and cover completely.

6. Carefully transfer the chicken to the stove and cook for 5-7 minutes on each side.

7. When you flip the chicken, add in the remaining ¼ cup of ghee and 1 tbsp thyme. Baste the chicken with the butter until fully cooked and golden.

8. Turn off the heat and add the tomato mixture back into the pan, then top with lemon juice.

9. Sprinkle fresh basil over top and serve right away.

23. Sweet Potato Pizza Crust with Spinach Pesto

Prep Time: 30 mins

Cook Time: 1 ½ hours

Total Time: 2 hours

Servings: 3

Ingredients

For the crust:

- 2 large sweet potatoes
- 1 clove garlic
- 1 tablespoon chia seeds
- 3 tablespoons water
- 1 1/4 cup gluten free oat flour
- 1/2 cup almond flour
- 1 tablespoon melted coconut oil
- 1 tablespoon apple cider vinegar
- 1 teaspoon dried oregano
- 1 teaspoon thyme

For the spinach pesto:

- 3 cups spinach

- 1 cup basil

- 3-4 tablespoons olive oil

- 2 cloves garlic

For the toppings:

- 1 onion + olive oil for caramelizing

- 1 cup cherry tomatoes

Instructions

1. Preheat oven to 400.

2. Use a fork to poke holes in sweet potatoes. Drizzle some coconut oil over sweet potatoes and 3 garlic cloves, and roast in oven for around 45 minutes (until tender).

3. Prepare chia egg by combining chia seeds and water. Let sit for 10 minutes.

4. Peel sweet potatoes and combine with garlic, gluten free oat flour, almond flour,coconut oil,apple cider vinegar,dried oregano and thyme.

5. Add the chia egg and mix.

6. Spread out the pizza crust on a parchment-paper lined oven tray.

7. Bake in 400 degree oven for about 30 minutes.

8. In processor,mix spinach, basil, olive oil and garlic to create thick pesto sauce.

9. Cut onion into thin slivers. Caramelize onion in pan for about 20 minutes (with olive oil on low heat).

10. Roast halved cherry tomatoes in 300 degree oven for 30 minutes until soft.

11. Add toppings onto pizza crust and cook for additional 10 minutes.

24. Summer Melon Salad with Prosciutto & Mozzarella

Prep Time: 20 mins

Cook Time: N/A

Total Time: N/N

Servings: 4

Ingredients

For the salad:

- 1 galia melon, seeded

- 1 orange honeydew, seeded

- 1 8oz container mozzarella balls (I used the ciliegine size)

- ¼ cup fresh basil leaves, thinly sliced

- 6 slices of prosciutto, torn into bite sized pieces

- For the lemon-honey dressing:
- 1 large lemon

- 2 teaspoon honey

- 1 teaspoon extra virgin olive oil

- Salt & pepper, to taste

Instructions

1. To make the vinaigrette: whisk all ingredients together until honey completely dissolves. Set aside while you prepare the salad.

2. To make the salad: Using a melon baller, scoop out small balls of the galia melon and honeydew and place in a large bowl.

3. Add the mozzarella balls and basil leaves.
4. Drizzle with vinaigrette, add prosciutto pieces.
5. Sprinkle with the rest of your basil and serve immediately.

25. Zesty Tomato, Arugula and Salami Pasta

Prep Time: 15 mins

Cook Time: 15 mins

Total Time: 30 mins

Servings: 4

Ingredients

- 4 cups gluten free pasta

- 2 tablespoons garlic infused olive oil

- 1 cup FODMAP-free salami (chopped)

- 1 large red pepper (diced)

- 1 teaspoon chilli flakes (dried)

- 3 large tomatoes (roughly chopped)

- 1 lemon (zested and juiced)

- 1 cup fresh parsley (chopped)

- ½ cup large handfuls of arugula

- salt to taste

- pepper to taste

- parmesan (optional)

Instructions

1. Cook pasta according to the instructions and drain well.
2. Meanwhile, in a large saucepan, heat 1 tablespoon of olive oil and fry the salami on a medium heat until it starts to become crispy.
3. Add peppers and fry both together for 3 minutes until the capsicum just starts to lose some of its crunch.
4. Add the chilli flakes and tomato and continue to fry until the tomato just starts to soften.
5. Add the lemon zest and juice. The juice should help to lift all the extra flavours from the pan.
6. Stir in cooked pasta, parsley and arugula and gently toss through until well combined.
7. Check seasoning and add salt and pepper if required.
8. Serve topped with freshly shaved parmesan.

26. BBQ Tempeh and Pineapple Skewers

Prep Time: 30 mins

Cook Time: 12 mins

Total Time: 42 mins

Servings: 4

Ingredients

- 1 package of tempeh

- 1 bottle of your favorite BBQ sauce (check the label to keep it gluten-free)

- 2 cups pineapple

- 2 bell peppers

- 1 large zucchini

- 1 small red onion

- 2 tablespoons avocado or olive oil

- wooden skewers

Instructions

1. To prep the tempeh: start by slicing the block into large pieces and add to a large freezer bag or container.
2. Pour in about 1/2 cup of the BBQ sauce and toss to coat the tempeh. Place in the fridge for 30 minutes to marinate while you prep the other ingredients.
3. To prep the grain: if serving with a grain, boil the water and cook the as directed on the package. Cover and set aside when ready to keep warm.
4. To prep the veggies: wash and slice all of the remaining veggies and pineapple into large bite-sized pieces (you want them big enough that they won't break/fall off the skewers.
5. Warm up the grill or grill pan on medium-high heat.
6. To assemble the skewers: lightly wet the wooden skewers to prevent them from burning. Slide, in any order, the marinated tempeh, pineapple, and veggies onto a skewer leaving enough empty space at each end to pick it up. Place it on a dish and continue until all of the ingredients are used up. Brush each skewer with a little oil to prevent sticking to the grill.
7. To cook: place the skewers on the preheated grill or grill pan. You want a nice sear so you should hear a sizzle once the skewers are over the heat. Cook for about 5 minutes

and rotate. Continue rotating every 5 minutes until each side has been seared and the veggies are just slightly tender.

8. Serve warm over the grain with a side of BBQ for dipping!

27. Grilled Corn & Feta Salad

Prep Time: 5 mins

Cook Time: 10 mins

Total Time: 15 mins

Servings: 4

Ingredients

- Dressing Ingredients:
- Juice of one lime
- 1/4 teaspoon lime zest
- 1 teaspoon honey
- 2 tablespoons red wine vinegar
- 2 tablespoons olive oil
- 1/2 tablespoon honey dijon mustard
- Cracked Sea Salt
- Ground Black Pepper

Salad Components:

- 2 ears corn shucked
- 1/4-1/3 cup feta cheese

- 1/2 red bell pepper

- 1/4 sweet yellow onion

- 1/4 cup Banza rice, uncooked

- 1/2 avocado

- Parsley

Instructions

1. Dressing: Whisk all ingredients together and set aside.

2. Salad: Shuck and rinse the corn. Set grill to 475 and lay directly on the grates.

3. Cook for 8 minutes, rotating the corn every two minutes. Keep an eye on it, so it doesn't burn and lower the heat if you need to.

4. Remove from the grill and melt a little butter over each cobb.

5. Cut kernels from the cobb.

6. Dice the red pepper and sweet onion. Saute in a little olive oil for 5-7 minutes. I like mine crisp tender so cooked on the shorter side. You could also leave these ingredients raw if you prefer.

7. Dice the avocado into chunks.

8. Cook the Banza rice according to package instructions.

9. Add all of the salad components to a bowl. Pour the dressing over the salad, and gently fold all the ingredients to coat.

10. Refrigerate for 30 to 1 hour. Garnish with parsley, more freshly ground black pepper, and a touch more salt (if needed and to your liking).

28. Cast Iron Deep Dish Cauliflower Crust (Keto, Gluten-Free)

Prep Time: 20 mins

Cook Time: 40 mins

Total Time: 1 hour

Servings: 5

Ingredients

- 4 cups cauliflower rice

- 2 eggs

- 1/3 cup almond flour

- 1/3 cup panko crumbs

- Salt and pepper to taste

Instructions

1. First preheat your oven to 425 degrees.

2. Steam and release the moisture from the cauliflower rice. I bought the rice pre-made as I think it is easier and less

time consuming! You can either steam the cauliflower in a pot of water over medium to high heat for about 7 minutes OR place in a microwaveable safe dish and place in the microwave for about 4-5 minutes. Then, allow to cool for a few minutes and place the rice into a paper towel or clean dish cloth and squeeze out any excess moisture.

3. In a large bowl add ALL of the ingredients and mix until well combined.

4. Place your cast iron pan on medium to high heat and add about 2-3 tbsp. of olive oil. Allow to heat for about 1-2 minutes.

5. Add the cauliflower "dough" into the cast iron pan and then press down firmly using a large spoon or spatula!

6. Allow to cook over the stove top for about 10 minutes on medium heat.

7. While the cauliflower crust is cooking – I scrapped the edges a bit so they were completely stuck to the side of the cast iron pan.

8. After 10 minutes, place the cast iron into the oven and bake at 425 degrees for 20 minutes.

9. After 20 minutes, leaving the oven on, add your toppings to the crust.

10. Bake for another 10 minutes or so. For the last few minutes you can turn the oven to broil and allow the top to became a bit crisper!

11. Slice and serve! The first slice may be a bit tricky getting out of the cast iron, so I suggest using a spatula!

12. To reheat simply place under the broiler for about 3 minutes! Lasts up to one week in the fridge.

29. Quick & Easy Cheeseburger Salad

Prep Time: 15 mins

Cook Time: A/N

Total Time: A/N

Servings: 4

Ingredients

- 4 cups mixed lettuce, chopped

- 1 lb ground beef

- Salt and pepper, to taste

- 1 cup grape tomatoes, sliced

- ½ red onion, finely chopped

- ⅓ cup cheddar cheese, grated

- Handful of dill pickles, quartered

- 2 tablespoons thousand island dressing

- For the croutons:

- 4-6 slices of your favorite bread, hamburger or hot dog buns

- Oil spray

- Salt

Instructions

1. To make the salad: Heavily season the ground beef with salt and pepper. Saute it until it's cooked all the way through. Set aside to cool.
2. In a large bowl, add the lettuce, tomatoes, red onion, pickles, cheese and ground beef after it's cooled.
3. Mix everything together. Drizzle with dressing right before you serve and top with any additional toppings
4. To make the croutons: Preheat oven to 375 degrees and line a baking sheet with parchment paper.
5. Cut the bread into 1 inch cubes and place them in a bowl. Spray the pieces with your oil spray until they're completely coated.
6. Sprinkle these pieces with salt and any other spices to your liking. Mix everything together and pour onto your prepared baking sheet.

7. Bake for 10 minutes or until the croutons are slightly brown.

8. When done, let them sit for a few minutes to harden as they cool.

30. Tuna Sashimi with Avocado Salad

Prep Time: 10 mins

Cook Time: N/A

Total Time: N/A

Servings: 2

Ingredients

- 1 tablespoon olive oil
- 1/2 teaspoon sesame oil
- 1 tablespoon tamari
- 1 tablespoon rice vinegar
- a dash of wasabi
- 175 g fillet of fresh tuna, cut into thin slices

FOR THE SALAD

- 1 avocado, sliced
- 8 cherry tomatoes, halved
- 2 heaped tablespoons freshly torn cilantro
- 3 spring onions, sliced
- juice of 1 lime
- sea salt and freshly ground black pepper
- 1 teaspoon toasted sesame seeds as garnish

Instructions

1. Pour the olive oil, sesame oil, tamari sauce and rice vinegar into a dish, then whisk in the wasabi. Add the tuna and coat well.
2. Layer the avocado, tomatoes, coriander and spring onions, squeeze over the lime juice and season to taste. Top with the dressed tuna and a sprinkling of sesame seeds.

31. Garlic Herb Biscuits

Prep Time: 10 mins

Cook Time: 13 mins

Total Time: 23 mins

Servings: 8

Ingredients

- 2 eggs

- 1/3 cup butter, melted

- 1/2 teaspoon salt

- 1/4 teaspoon black pepper

- 1/2 teaspoon basil

- 1/2 teaspoon garlic powder

- 1/2 teaspoon dried chives

- 2 teaspoon baking powder

- 2 cups almond flour

Instructions

1. Preheat your oven to 350F and line a baking sheet with parchment paper

2. Melt your butter in the microwave and set aside.

3. Get a large bowl and combine your almond flour, baking powder, and other spices

4. In another bowl mix your eggs and butter together! Then add in your dry ingredients

5. Combine dough well and form into 8 biscuits!

6. Bake for 13 minutes. Transfer to a cooling rack for a few minutes! DIG IN!

32. Chocolate Coconut Donuts (Paleo)

Prep Time: 10 mins

Cook Time: 10 mins

Total Time: 20 mins

Servings: 6

Ingredients

- 1/2 cup pumpkin puree

- 1/4 cup unsweetened applesauce

- 1/4 cup honey

- 1/4 cup buttermilk

- 1/4 teaspoon vanilla

- 1/4 cup milk

- 2 tablespoon baking powder

- 1/2 teaspoon baking soda

- 1 tablespoon cornstarch

- 2 tablespoon ground flaxseed

- 1/4 cup cocoa powder

- 1/3 cup spelt flour

- 1/4-1/2 cup white chocolate

- Unsweetened coconut flakes

Instructions

1. Preheat your oven to 375F
2. In a small bowl mix in your wet ingredients
3. Slowly add in your dry ingredients. Mix until incorporated
4. Grease your donut pans and scoop the batter into the pan
5. Bake for 10 minutes
6. Makes about 6 donuts
7. Once the donuts have cooled, dip them in the melted white chocolate and roll them into the coconut lakes (placed in a separate bowl)

33. Healthy Superfood Cookies

Prep Time: 10 mins

Cook Time: 20 mins

Total Time: 30 mins

Servings: 18 cookies

Ingredients

- 1 cup rolled oats

- 1/2 cup almond flour

- 1/4 cup flaxseed meal

- 1 tablespoon chia seeds

- 1/4 cup raw pumpkin seeds

- 1/4 cup sunflower seeds

- 1 teaspoon cinnamon

- 1/4 teaspoon salt

- 1/2 teaspoon baking powder

- 1/2 cup raisins

- 1/2 cup unsweetened applesauce

- 3 tablespoons melted coconut oil

- 3 tablespoons maple syrup

- 2 tablespoons almond milk

Instructions

1. Preheat the oven to 325°F and line a baking sheet with parchment paper.
2. In a large bowl add in all of the dry ingredients (oats, flour, nuts, seeds, dried fruit, salt, cinnamon, baking powder) and mix until combined.
3. Add in the applesauce, coconut oil, maple syrup, and almond milk. Mix until a sticky batter is formed.
4. Divide and roll the batter (about 1-2 tbsp of batter per cookie) into cookies (about 18 cookies).
5. Bake in the oven for 18-20 minutes or until the edges are golden brown. Let the cookies cool for a few minutes until transferring to a cooling rack for 10 minutes. Store in the refrigerator or freezer and enjoy!

34. Chickpea Chocolate Chip Cookies

Prep Time: 35 mins

Cook Time: 25 mins

Total Time: 1 hour

Servings: 12 cookies

Ingredients

- 1 15oz can chickpeas
- 1/2 cup almond butter creamy/smooth
- 3 tablespoons maple syrup
- 2 tablespoons coconut oil melted
- 1 teaspoons vanilla extract
- 2 1/2 tablespoons coconut sugar
- 3 tablespoons almond flour
- 1/4 teaspoon paleo baking powder
- 1/4 teaspoon baking soda
- 1/2 teaspoon salt
- 1/2 cup chocolate chips, add more if you want them extra chocolatey

Instructions

1. Line a baking sheet with parchment paper and preheat oven to 350°F. Drain and rinse the can of chickpeas.

2. Add all of the ingredients to a blender or food processor, leaving out the chocolate chips, and blend until you have a fairly smooth batter. Fold in the chocolate chips. Leave some out if you want to add some directly on top of the cookies before baking!

3. Place your dough in the refrigerator for 30-45 minutes to let it firm up a bit before forming into balls. You can transfer the cookie dough to a separate bowl or just place the blender in the refrigerator.

4. Once your dough is set, begin rolling the dough into balls and place on the cookie sheet. I like to wet my fingers after and then smooth down the tops of the cookies to make them have less stiff peaks. Add any additional chocolate chips.

5. Bake for 23-25 minutes or until the cookies are brown and a little firm on the outside. Once removed from the oven, let cool on the baking sheet for a bit before transferring to a cooling rack to cool completely.

6. I like to store these in the freezer as they are a gooier cookie but the refrigerator works as well! Enjoy!

35. Samoa Cookie Bars

Prep Time: 20 mins

Cook Time: 20 mins

Total Time: 40 mins

Servings: 16

Ingredients

- For the crust:
- 2/3 cup coconut flour
- pinch of salt
- 2 1/2 tablespoon maple syrup
- 1/3 cup coconut oil (solid)
- 6 tablespoons water
- For the filling:
- 1/2 cup creamy almond butter
- 1/3 cup maple syrup
- pinch of salt
- 1 teaspoon vanilla extract
- 3/4 cup dark chocolate dairy free
- 1/3 cup coconut oil

- 3/4 cup shredded coconut unsweetened

Instructions

For The Crust:

1. Preheat oven to 350°F and line an 8×8" square pan with parchment paper and grease the inside edges.
2. In a bowl, combine the coconut flour and salt. Add the maple syrup, coconut oil, and water until well combined. If the mixture is still too crumbly, add water, a tbsp at a time, until a dough forms.
3. In the prepared pan, press the dough into an even layer and bake for approximately 16-17 minutes or until the edges are golden. Set aside to cool.

For The Filling:

1. In a small saucepan, combine the almond butter, maple syrup, coconut oil, vanilla, and salt. Heat the mixture until it is completely melted and combined.
2. Pour the mixture over the crust and then sprinkle the shredded coconut all over the top. Place in the

refrigerator to set. After it is set, you can cut into 16 squares.

3. Melt half of the dark chocolate in the microwave and stir until smooth. Take each square and dip the bottom into the melted chocolate and place on a lined baking sheet to set.

4. Melt the rest of the chocolate in the microwave. Pour the chocolate into a ziplock bag and snip the corner off. Squeeze the bag to drizzle over all of the squares for decoration.

5. Store in refrigerator or freezer and enjoy!

36. Chocolate Rose Energy Balls (Vegan)

Prep Time: 10 mins

Cook Time: 20 mins

Total Time: 30 mins

Servings: 12

Ingredients

- 5 fresh, pitted dates smashed & diced

- 1 cup almond flour

- 1/2 cup dark chocolate sunflower seed butter (or favorite nut butter)

- 1/4 cup pure maple syrup

- 1/4 cup oat flour

- 1 tsp cardamom

- 1 tsp food grade rosewater

- 1/4 cup goji berries

- 1/4 cup chopped vegan chocolate chunks

Instructions 95

1. Start with a large bowl. Chop up and mash the dates well so they can easily be incorporated. I left a few chunks because I like a more chunky bliss ball.
2. Add in the almond flour, and chocolate sun butter, mix well.
3. Add maple syrup, oat flour, cardamom & rosewater. Mix until very well combined.
4. Fold in the goji berries and chocolate shreds.
5. Roll into balls, place on a baking sheet & put in the freezer for about 30 minutes.
6. Store in fridge & ENJOY!

37. Bacon-Wrapped Jalapeno Poppers

Prep Time: 15 mins

Cook Time: 20 mins

Total Time: 35 mins

Servings: 15

Ingredients

- 3-4 jalapenos sliced into rounds

- 1 lb bacon strips uncooked

- 8 oz plain cream cheese

- 1 lb shrimp frozen, cooked OR fresh, uncooked

- 1 tablespoon sriracha

- Black pepper to taste

- Chili powder to taste

Instructions

1. Preheat your smoker to 225 degrees Fahrenheit (or normal grill to medium-high heat).
2. Slice jalapenos into ~1/4 inch thick rounds, and cut bacon strips in half.
3. Spread 1-2 tsp of cream cheese on to the top of each jalapeno slice.
4. Lay the cream cheese-covered jalapeno slice on the end of one piece of bacon.
5. Top jalapeno & cream cheese slice with a piece of shrimp. Roll the bacon strip over the wrap it tightly into a "roll" and stick a toothpick through each one to keep it secure.
6. Repeat until ingredients are gone.
7. Transfer all of your bacon-wrapped jalapeno poppers to preheated grill and cook for roughly 18-20 minutes or until bacon is cooked to your liking. Flip halfway through. (Check temperature of shrimp before removing if using fresh, uncooked shrimp. Should be cooked to internal temp of 145 degrees F.)
8. Enjoy hot off the grill!
9. Store leftovers in an airtight container in the fridge for 2-3 days.

38. Raw Vegan Brownie Bites

Prep Time: 15 mins

Cook Time: N/A

Total Time: N/A

Servings: 8

Ingredients

- 1 cup cashews

- 1 cup pitted dates

- 2 tablespoons coconut nectar

- 1 tablespoon coconut oil

- ½ cup cacao powder

- 1 tablespoon lucuma

- 1 tablespoon vanilla extract

- ¼ teaspoon salt

- 1 cup of almonds, walnuts, or pistachios

Instructions

1. Place the cashews in a food processor and pulse into small pieces.
2. Add in dates, coconut nectar, coconut oil, cacao powder, lucuma, vanilla extract, and salt and process until well mixed.
3. Add ¾ cup of the nut of your choice and pulse into mixture until pieces are chopped up.
4. Roll mixture into individual 'bites,' about 1 ½ inches in diameter.
5. Use the remaining ¼ cup of nuts, chopped, and roll the brownie bites on the chopped nuts to add nuts to the outside.

39. Dried Plum and Pistachio Chia Pudding

Prep Time: 5 mins

Cook Time: 60 mins

Total Time: 1 hour 5 mins

Servings: 2

Ingredients

- 1/3 cup chia seeds
- 1 1/2 cups unsweetened almond milk (or other non-dairy milk)
- 1/2 cup California Dried Plums (chopped) + additional for topping
- 1/3 cup pistachios roasted + additional for topping
- 2 tablespoons hemp seeds
- 1 tablespoon cacao nibs unsweetened + additional for topping
- 2 teaspoon cinnamon ground

Instructions

1. Whisk together ingredients in large mixing bowl.

2. Cover and chill in fridge for at least one hour or overnight.

3. Once mixture reaches a pudding-like consistency, remove from fridge and divide into 2 bowls or mason jars.

4. Top with additional chopped California Dried Plums, pistachios, and cacao nibs before serving.

40. Mixed Berry & Tahini Chia Pudding

Prep Time: 5 mins

Cook Time: 10 mins

Total Time: 15 mins

Servings: 4

Ingredients

- 1 cup frozen mixed berries (I used a combination of strawberries, blueberries & blackberries)

- 1 cup canned organic coconut milk

- 1/2 cup unsweetened almond or milk of preference

- 1/4 cup Further Food Vanilla Collagen
- 1/4 cup tahini

- 1 teaspoon pure vanilla extract

- Sugar-free monk fruit sweetener, pure stevia, or sweetener of choice, adjusted to taste

- 1/2 cup chia seeds

Instructions

1. Put frozen berries, coconut milk, almond or nut-free milk, collagen or protein, tahini, and vanilla into blender container and blend well. Sweeten to taste.
2. Add chia seeds and pulse blend until just combined.
3. Pour into a bowl or single-serving mason jars and cover or seal tightly.
4. Let sit for 10 minutes, then shake or whisk well and put in fridge overnight or for a minimum of 4 hours.
5. Mixed Berry & Tahini Chia Pudding can be stored in an airtight container in the fridge for 4 to 5 days. Serve warm or cold with your choice of toppings.

www.ingramcontent.com/pod-product-compliance
Lightning Source LLC
Chambersburg PA
CBHW070813170726
48000CB00017B/881